TABLE OF CONTENTS

AUTHOR CREDENTIALS

Margaret Phalor Barnhart is a graduate of:
Capital University, Columbus, OH, 1962 BS in Education
Miami University, Oxford, OH, 1970 ME Guidance & Counseling
Wright State University, Dayton, OH, 1988 Masters of Art Therapy

M.P. Barnhart had 17 years as teacher and elementary school counselor throughout Ohio

Author: Journey Unknown, 2nd Edition, 2012
Contributor to books and magazine articles

2014 Winner of "Words of Inspiration," American Breast Care competition.

Member of Christ Community Church
2015 Commissioned as a Stephen Minister

Lives in Tucson, Arizona with husband Charlie

For speaking engagements contact her by

Email: margeb730@cox.net
Website: www.margaretbarnhart.com

TRIBUTES

"The best compliment I can pay to Marge Barnhart and her writings - and I have read and distributed scores in my clinical visits to Cancer Patients and their Care Providers - is that her works are pertinent, holistically-relative and caring. The two sides of the author: her personal walk through the cancer process and her biblical relevance has made her a tender-loving, caring survivor, counselor, and mentor. Barnhart writes not in a 'braggadocios' manner of any sort, but as a fellow-traveler, empathizing with the challenges of cancer, yet presenting an unshakable trust in the providence of God."

Carl H. Smith, PHD

Serving the Lord through Biblical teaching, mercy and compassion at the back door of Europe (Romania)

LaVerne writes,

"I have said these things to you, that in me
you may have peace. In the world you will
have tribulation. But take heart; I have
overcome the world." John 16:33

"In a penetrating writing style, Margaret
Phalor Barnhart allows the reader to become
intimate with her story and those of five other
courageous people afflicted with a variety of
cancers.

In the face of fearful reality and sometimes
overwhelming circumstances, each shares
their struggle against this threatening disease.
Their stories are inspirational, and their
victories are a testament to the overcoming
power of faith, hope, and fortitude."

Nurses from Arizona Oncology write,

"Easy, light-hearted read. Good endeavor at capturing and revealing the spectrum of cancer care and the daily challenges each patient and family go through while living with cancer.

The author has grasped many natural human honest experiences while trying to reveal the truth of living with cancer. The balance of details varies throughout the book depending on each individual experience. Some of the experiences left me wanting more.

The author displays a passion toward patients living with cancer on a topic that remains taboo, to others who have not been touched by the disease.

 Enjoyed reading."

PREFACE

Driving east on Speedway Blvd. the heavy downpour gradually lessened and the sun peeked through the clouds. The sun was off to my right, rear side of the car. When I looked to the left I saw the first glimmer of a rainbow.

Dark clouds on the other side of the fully formed rainbow intensified the colors. The clouds were the source of the storm.

A diagnosis of cancer creates a storm. No matter how gently the doctor makes the announcement an individual is shocked. Although we appear to be listening, it is common to go off into space and not hear the rest of what is said.

Many years ago cancer was a death sentence. In the late 1940s my father, at the age of 30, was diagnosed with Hodgkin's disease. The doctor told my mother to prepare for her husband's death. However, x-ray treatments (radiation) worked and Dad lived an active life for 40 years.

The stories in this book are true and I am most appreciative of those who shared their personal experience with cancer. Some people I asked to participate by telling their story chose not to discuss their experience, similar to those who have gone to war and returned home. I loved when Jack said to me, "I don't want to upset you, but who would want to read this stuff?"

My goal in bringing these stories to light is to give you, the reader, an inside look at cancer from different perspectives. No two experiences are the same. No two people with the same diagnosis are the same. A treatment for one may not work for another.

The feelings expressed in the stories are universal but will differ in intensity. Reactions to those feelings will also differ. Diagnosis, treatment, age, and circumstances will bring different results.

Reading this book will expose you to an understanding that hope exists. Spirituality will play a part as well as specific religious beliefs.

The contributors have been diagnosed with various forms of cancer; including lung, bladder, metastases following breast cancer, prostate, cancer of the tongue, and the author's breast cancer. A high percentage of people who have been diagnosed with cancer are alive and functioning in the world today.

Margaret Phalor Barnhart
Christian Author and Editor

CRYSTAL

LUNG CANCER

AGE 61
when diagnosed

CRYSTAL -- LUNG CANCER

I am a cancer survivor and my story begins toward the end of the year 2000 when my husband and I moved from Dayton, NV to Tucson, AZ. We were still unpacking when our good friends and RV travel buddies from Chico, CA stopped by for a visit early in January, 2001. They were on their way to Kino Bay in Mexico, through the Nogales, Sonora, Mexico Port of Entry.

The Border Patrol stopped them to search their pickup. Carol's husband forgot that he had a rifle stored in the back of his pickup. This put an immediate halt to their travel plans as the rifle was confiscated, along with their pickup truck and motor home, and he was taken to jail.

Carol had no choice but to spend the night in Nogales, Sonora. I drove down the next day to pick her up and bring her to our home in Tucson. The one way trip took an hour and a half. Then to get to the prison we had to park and take a taxi. Every day we drove from Tucson to Nogales to visit her husband in prison. It was March 2001 when he was released.

During that stressful time I developed a cough but was busy helping our friends and didn't seek medical care. (After all, it was just a cough.) Once the friends returned to Chico, I realized I did need to be seen. However, as a newcomer to Tucson I had no established doctor. It was difficult to find one who accepted new patients.

In early April, 2001, I was able to see a nurse practitioner who said many people contract Valley Fever when they come to Tucson. To rule that out it was necessary to do blood work and have x-rays taken. Later that same day, the doctor called and said there was a mass in my left lung, the size of an egg. That was a jolt!

 Thus began the journey of having biopsies, CT scans, PET scans and finally seeing an oncologist who said at age 61 I was young enough and healthy enough to be treated aggressively.

After twenty-two radiation treatments and four chemotherapy sessions I became very fatigued and had difficulty sleeping. I was advised to sit in a warm tub of water and drink black tea.

In August the decision was made to have the lump surgically removed. I was notified that the doctor scheduled to perform the surgery, broke his arm while on vacation with his son--skate boarding. He had a cast on his arm and he supervised as his associate removed the top lobe of my left lung where the tumor was located.

I was expected to go home from the hospital in three or four days. Ten days later I was still there because the surgical site continued to drain.

The post surgery report indicated the tissue surrounding the mass was free of cancer. Lymph nodes were cancer free. I was told that if there was a relapse, it typically happens within the first two years.

Sunday Aug 26, 2001. Thank you, God, for bringing me through this. What a wonder to be home. Being in the hospital with all the tubes becomes tiresome. The bed and pillow never fit right. Now I can have my own bed and my own pillow.

I had pain in the surgery site and where the tube came out on my left side. There was also pain in my back. I wasn't feeling well. The doctor ordered pain medication and that helped.

Several days later I went to the mall and walked around. That was tiring. No one told me how to behave after all these treatments.

October 10 and I still experience pain in my back and left side near my breast. I took a bath in moisturizers. Every morning I cough but am still walking on a regular basis. I went a mile today. I thought I would be much better by now.

November came and I went to a support group meeting. I had an appointment to see my pulmonologist. He wanted to know if I was using my inhalers. Yes. Since there were no more symptoms I didn't make any more appointments with him.

I was having trouble sleeping through the night. What are these funny noises in my left chest area? I made an appointment to see my oncologist who said x-rays are OK and now he has a baseline for future reference. The blood work showed anemia but that was cleared up before my second blood draw.

A CT scan was ordered for two months from now. Funny noises? Who knows? Every once in a while I wake up with intense pain in my left breast area and then find it hard to get back to sleep.

It is early December and I feel stressed about birthdays and Christmas. My husband's mother moved in and stayed with us for the next six months. That too was stressful. She ultimately spent 3 years in various nursing homes.

I have survived. I am no longer a lung cancer patient and am now involved with support groups and am pursuing ways to help with early detection. People often ask me if I smoke/smoked.

My answer to that question is yes, I did. However, I stopped 17 years prior to being diagnosed. Why do people ask that question? It makes me feel that I am responsible. Maybe my years of smoking did lead me to a cancer diagnosis. However, second-hand smoke and the environment can also cause lung cancer. If you have lungs, you can get lung cancer.

More women are being diagnosed with lung cancer than men. Early detection is critical. An early symptom often presents as a dry cough. I will continue my quest to promote early detection and knowledge about lung cancer.

JACK

BLADDER
CANCER

Age 70
when diagnosed

JACK – BLADDER CANCER

Born in 1920, a boy named Jack came into the world during the Depression. His home was in Milwaukee, Wisconsin.

It was a small house on the West side of the city. Some would say that was the poor folk's neighborhood.

The Foundry was the place where many men worked. It was difficult to find a job anywhere.

Jack left home after graduating from high school to fight in World War II. He was drafted into the Army Air Corp and worked as an instructor who trained with pilots both on simulated equipment and in the air. Although not a certified pilot, he could take over the plane if necessary.

Now he thinks it was stupid, but he became a four pack a day cigarette smoker. Following his time in the military he went back home to live with his parents in their one bedroom house.

He worked some in the Foundry and began a college education at the University of Wisconsin extension in Milwaukee and completed the two year liberal arts program.

Jack also worked for the Republican Party, helping the governor by setting up speaker systems. He was paid $14.00 a week. The Governor won the election and that left Jack unemployed.

Next Jack worked for the Falk Company. They manufactured various size gears from small to huge. His job was to be a time keeper and produce reports on the time it took to do a job. He enrolled in the School of Management at Northwestern.

After two and a half years he graduated in May, 1949. He now had two degrees, one in Production Management and one in Personnel Administration.

Jack's mother had a job as a clerk and knew a young woman she wanted him to meet. After all, he was thirty-one years old and still living with his parents.

It took a lot of nerve and Jack felt out of place because this girl lived on the east side of Milwaukee. In other words, she was from a family that had much more money than Jack's family. The age difference also concerned him. He was 31 and she was 23.

Nevertheless they began dating and really liked each other. For Christmas he gave her an engagement ring and they married in April, 1951 and were together for more than 60 years.

His wife's father was President of Pabst Brewing Company while Jack worked for the Steel Corporation. Steel was bought out by the Falk Corporation. Jack was given a job there and with his experience and education he quickly moved up the ladder to management. He became known for preventing the Falk Corporation from becoming unionized. He soon moved up to Vice-President.

He and his wife had two children, both girls. They and their mother went to church, but he wasn't interested. In fact, he was 85 years old before he became a church go-er and was baptized.

In the year 1990 at the age of 70, Jack was noticing he had to void urine more frequently. He was referred to an urologist (who happened to be a friend) and a Cystoscopy was performed.

"The Cystoscopy can examine the entire bladder area. The doctor uses a thin, lighted tube that can be inserted through the urethra and into the bladder. A small video camera is at the tip, allowing the doctor to see inside. Sterile salt water is injected through the Cystoscope, which expands the bladder, making it easier to examine." (WebMD.com)

His friend gently told him he had cancer of the bladder. At first he panicked. This was a whole new world that opened up to him--and not one of which he wanted to be a part.

Realizing he had a choice--treatment or no treatment, he chose the treatment. His wife was by his side. Jack's urologist friend retired so he began treatment with a new urologist.

For an extended time he went into the office where a tube was inserted into the penis and a liquid was injected. It reached a point when they all agreed that he would stop treatment. He was evaluated every three months.

Recurrence!

That is a word no one wants to hear. This time it was decided that removing part of the bladder was the best choice. The doctor drew pictures so Jack had a better understanding of what he was facing. The date was set. He was on the gurney outside the operating room when his pastor hurried to his side and the two of them, along with the surgeon, prayed for a good outcome.

Following the surgery, it was necessary to remove blood clots. That involved placing a catheter to deliver a clot-busting liquid. This was an extremely painful procedure and Jack found himself yelling in pain--definitely not a nice man's grunt!

Life returned to normal and the golf matches were a source of pleasure. A year later, the cancer was back and Jack was referred to an oncologist. He began chemotherapy. He was ready to die, but agreed to try a new treatment that involved infusion.

Walking into the infusion room was a shock in its own way. There sat four rows of women in lounge chairs with five or six women in each row. They were all connected to tubes. He was the only man.

Jack was given an injection of medication to combat nausea and after fifteen minutes the chemotherapy agents began and lasted fifty minutes. At first all was well. Then his blood count changed and he felt terrible.

The infusions went on for eight weeks. Jack was appalled that the medication cost $8,000 a week. It was covered by insurance. And, he didn't lose his hair!

Next in the treatment plan was radiation that was aimed at his bladder and hip bones. This took 30 sessions once a week. Bladder cancer left Jack with two-thirds of his bladder and weakness in his legs. He no longer has the strength to golf.

Jack and his wife travelled to various sites in Arizona. His wife enjoyed teaching children true Indian stories.

Jack is now in his 90's. His wife died several years ago.

Tests show a spot in one area of his lung but there is no plan to treat it. He has great neighbors and friends, likes going to church and treats himself to one shot of Scotch a day!

LINDA

BREAST CANCER WITH RECURRENCE OF INVASIVE DUCTAL CARCINOMA AND METASTASES

Age 52 when diagnosed

LINDA -- BREAST CANCER WITH RECURRENCE OF INVASIVE DUCTAL CARCINOMA AND METASTASES

In August of 2011, I was diagnosed with invasive ductal carcinoma in my left breast and a "suspicious mass" in my right breast.

I had two mammograms, x-rays, an ultra-sound guided biopsy and an MRI. My breasts were purple, black and blue from all the probing. My diagnosis changed to bilateral breast carcinoma with different subtypes.

I was really missing my husband John, my rock, my faith reminder, my love, John who always assured me, "Everything will be OK." If he was still alive, I wouldn't need to turn to anyone else.

I am left with my thoughts...What is cancer? Is it real? Can it really harm me? In my lifetime of practicing my faith, there is one thing I know for sure that God is the only Creator and He created Good. All else is not real, rather temporary, a dream perhaps, like the "Adam dream" in Genesis from which he never awoke. I'm trying to balance my thoughts and my worlds, Spiritual and physical. Almost without thinking about it, I close my eyes and repeat the verse I learned so well.

"There is no life, truth, intelligence, nor substance in matter. All is infinite Mind and its infinite manifestation, for God is All-in-all.
"Spirit is immortal Truth; matter is mortal error. Spirit is the real and eternal; matter is the unreal and temporal.
"Spirit is God, and man is His image and likeness. Therefore man is not material; he is spiritual."

Science and Health with Key to the Scriptures by Mary Baker Eddy, page 468

Thank you, God.

My decision to have a double mastectomy in September 2011 was made quickly; taking into account my family history and a myriad of other thoughts. I wasn't surprised or scared or upset.

I had felt the lump even before John died. I was busy with teaching, taking care of the household and attending to John's needs.

After he passed from this earth in 2007, I focused on teaching and was preparing for retirement. I couldn't be bothered with my medical issues; there were other things that grabbed my attention.

The diagnosis was something to move past, to get over. I remember thinking that this was the way for me to get the "perfect boobs" I always wanted. Insurance would pay for surgeries and reconstruction because it wouldn't be "cosmetic;" rather cancer. Was I really that superficial?? I always thought I looked past the book's cover and here I am doing it to myself. Hmmmm...Fodder for much thought!!!

Because I was so focused on "new boobs" I did not educate myself about the surgery and the recovery. The immediate post-surgery seemed to be going well; nothing out of the ordinary. I was in the hospital overnight, released the next day with drains pinned to my t-shirt and mega bandages over the place where my breasts used to be. I was surprised at the amount of bandages, the huge scars and the inability to use my arms during recovery.

My sister came from Wisconsin to stay with me for a week and I was very glad she was here. I couldn't lift the jug of milk, or the pot to make soup; or, drive my car for two months! After that week, other loved ones came over to help me because I was still a lump in a chair or in bed, with my arms propped up on pillows along-side me.

My surgeon pronounced me "cured" a week later and presented me with a little pink beach sandal. She removed the left drain and said, "Let me know when the draining of fluid on the right side has lessened and you are ready for it to come out."

Teaching was always on my mind. I was feeling pretty good, so I informed my principal I would be returning. He was thrilled. However on my first day back I ended up leaving mid-day because I was bleeding through my bandages, onto my clothing.

I continued to bleed and called the surgeon's office for advice. I was told to apply pressure.

The next day I demanded to see my surgeon because something was wrong. She discovered I had an eight centimeter tunnel in my right side that needed a wound vacuum to heal.

It became apparent that I would not be returning to school anytime soon. In order to qualify for home nursing I needed to remain home-bound.

The nurse came to my house every other day to remove old sponges and tubes. She used an extra-long Q-tip to clean and measure the tunnel. Then she replaced sterile sponges and affixed the wound vacuum to new tubes. This procedure continued for three months.

My students had a month with me as their teacher at the beginning of the school year and prior to my surgery. I worried about school. My third grader's learning was being disrupted by having a variety of substitutes.

I wanted to provide as much consistency as possible so I continued to write lesson plans and grade papers at home. Colleagues graciously brought me student papers. This turned out to be harder than I expected--typing and writing with only my left hand because the right side was still healing.

I believed I was cheating my students; however, I, their teacher needed time to recuperate. I went back to work a week before Christmas break, after the right breast incision healed.

The children were happy to see me and the feeling was mutual. However, before long I found myself becoming fatigued before the day ended and my patience grew short. Six months to go until the end of the year and my retirement.

The surgeon said I was now ready to talk about prosthetics. The American Cancer Society has a sharing center where individuals can receive free services and supplies. The prostheses I chose were foam and sewn into a bra. It was fairly comfortable, but I looked for a different type because of the heat of a Tucson summer!!

My doctor wrote a prescription for silicone prosthetics and a special bra that my insurance covered. I also ordered a pair of micro-bead, light-weight prosthetics from the American Cancer Society Website – Tender Loving Care (TLC), as well as numerous undergarments to encase my new "not" breasts.

Anticipating my retirement in June, 2012 I had been researching travel agencies, tour groups and the like for about a year. I found the perfect group.

I settled on traveling with Singles Travel International. They had fair rates and I could have a room for myself, paying a slight increase rather than double the cost as most tours do. As I would be traveling with prosthetics I was uncomfortable with the idea of having a roommate. Privacy was essential. I decided the foam looked best and packed the micro-beads as back-ups.

IRELAND--here I come.

I left Tucson on April 26th, 2013, almost a year after my school retirement, choosing the foam prostheses to wear on the plane. They have metal cores so going through security could be a challenging experience.

After placing all of my belongings and shoes in the x-ray bins, I walked toward the screening archway. I moved forward as directed by security personnel and when the alarm went off, I was ushered to a private security room. I told the guard that I was wearing breast prostheses and they have a metal core. She used the wand over my body and thanked me for my cooperation. I was excused. It was a fairly quick detour and not at all invasive. Now I know the routine and was okay with it.

The itinerary was Tucson to Philadelphia to Dublin--eight days and seven nights of exploring green hills and countryside of Dublin one night; Galway City two nights; Killarney two nights; then back to Dublin for two more nights. This was a most memorable trip and I have 500 photos from 20 major sites to facilitate my memory. I loved Ireland and was busy looking at everything and taking in all the information my brain could possibly handle.

There were a couple of days that I chose the micro-bead prostheses because they were comfortable and I thought they would hold up better in the rain that had been predicted. I didn't want to get the foam boobs wet. It would take forever for them to dry out! Funny, huh!! I was happy to have my own room, my private space, to take them off and relax.

Going through security was not a problem the rest of the trip. I would love to visit beautiful Ireland again.

Arriving home on May 4th, I needed about a week to come back to earth and get all my travel treasures sorted out. Now it was time to coordinate my Bozeman, MT and Las Vegas, NV trips. The plan was to fly to Bozeman for a visit with friends, and then continue on to Las Vegas.

MONTANA

Montana's beauty first struck me at the Bozeman Airport--huge log beams and beautiful earth colors. The outdoors is amazing in May, green everywhere and mild temperatures. My friends, Steve and Kanella, live in a log cabin on acres of sky-high trees, clear streams and the Galatin River.

One day we drove to Yellowstone National Park, passing rushing rivers and snowy mountains. The trip to Ireland and now this time in Montana broadened my focus and took it off cancer. No one noticed I had a bi-lateral mastectomy. After strapping on the fake boobs, and clothing my body, I looked like every other woman. I have been struggling with my new body image and cry a lot.

One morning I sleepily got out of bed, not thinking about where I was, and emerged into the main part of the cabin in my PJ's. When I realized I was boob-less I quickly covered up with a sweatshirt. Steve left for work, apparently not paying attention to me. Kanella and I were alone when the "flood gates" opened, allowing my tears to flow. She and I had good girlfriend talk.

That was the first time anyone saw me without boobs or the appearance of boobs. Is that being fake? Having fake boobs? Symbolic twist! I viewed myself as no longer normal. Things had changed. I believed I needed to "act as if" everything was fine when it wasn't. Is that being positive or foolish?

Nature is all around and this place is a wonderful location to meditate and clear the mind. I spent time down by the stream thinking, crying and talking to God. The sky is a brilliant blue. I can hear the birds. I have Love and feel so blessed. Thank you, God.

I guess each moment has its own reality. I have a choice how to feel from moment to moment. To say I have bouts of sadness and a feeling of deformity is true, but I eventually return to my faith. There I find peace, comfort, purpose and the only thing I know for sure! That God, Good, is the only power at work in my life. Things go so well when I remember this! I left Montana entertaining the thought of breast reconstruction. I should at least have a consultation.

LAS VEGAS, NV

My next stop on this summer's travel is to Las Vegas, Nevada. The plan is to meet friends from Flagstaff and go to their granddaughter's first birthday celebration. I had a reservation at the Palace Station Casino mostly because of location.

The rooms in this hotel were well appointed and I felt pampered just by the decor. I enjoyed time alone, getting my thoughts clear. I did some internet research on reconstruction and spent more time crying.

I left Las Vegas thinking how to love my body the way it is. Really, wearing prosthetics feels like misrepresenting myself--unreal--not me. I had lots of time for research and firmly decided I did not want reconstruction. I don't want to have drains all over again!!

I'm home now in Tucson, in my new apartment, going through all my travel memories. It has been an amazing few months--First Ireland, then majestic Montana, and lastly Las Vegas. There is a great deal to process and digest.

In the years that followed, I lived a semi-retired life, working part-time in a variety of roles including substituting at "my school." Before long I found myself with less energy and patience to teach a full day. I was thankful because I was retired I didn't have to do more than I could manage.

It is toward the end of 2013 and I still struggle whether or not to wear prosthetics. I heard from one woman that, "it was not professional and obviously I didn't care about the way I looked."

Making my decision, I put the special bras and various prostheses in a drawer so they were available if I ever changed my mind. Frankly, I am much more comfortable in my own skin and can walk with dignity.

Today I have my copper—sparkled, ruffled swimsuit on with no prosthetics. The ruffles are on top and my flat chest is not noticeable.

Walking through the apartment complex I thought about who I might see. "Stop walking with your head down, Linda," I told myself. I stood erect and confident as I walked the winding sidewalk. When I arrived, I saw I was the only swimmer--nobody but me.

I walked into the pool, stretched my ankles and calf muscles and began my swim routine. Breast strokes, proper breast strokes, then freestyle, achieving a great stretch with each stroke. I didn't feel out of balance, actually it felt good to just be myself.

After drying in the morning sun, I turned over to get a little exposure for the back of my legs. I couldn't lie down completely; my chest hurt. The combination of the increased exercise and Cocoa Butter regimen are leaving a bit of soreness across my chest and under my arms. I rested on my elbows just long enough so I wouldn't be dripping for the walk home.

I'm talking to myself the whole way home, affirming the evidence of why I should be confident. "You are wise," I said to myself. That's what John would say.

I looked up. The sky was a brilliant blue. I could hear birds. I have choices. I have Love and I am so blessed! Thank you God!

MAY, 2015 **RECURRENCE!**

I noticed small lumps on the scar from my left breast that I would not have noticed had I chosen reconstruction. The diagnosis was recurrent breast cancer and metastasis to the lung lining (pleura.) I anticipated what I was told, but I worried about how to tell my mom.

Growing up, Mom taught me to seek God first to know the truth. In 2011 when I told her about the diagnosis she forgot all teachings and I had to remind her about our faith.

Now in 2015 when I told her about the recurrence she cried and asked what the doctor said. It didn't take her long to reach her long held beliefs. Thinking back I realized that I left God out of the treatment plan the first time around and now, this time, we would be partners.

I was now restricted from any type of work. Massive amounts of co-pays, tests and drug costs were prohibitive. With the help of an attorney I filed for Social Security Disability. It was approved because of the new diagnosis. Now the stress and worry of paying for my medical treatment was lifted.

Knowing that all wisdom comes from Him, my doctor would be guided by His wisdom. Those who practice medicine are also guided by God. I need to remember this. It is important to me because I truly want to know how Spiritual healing and physical (earthly) comfort complement each other--the best of both worlds.

Once more I know that God is an ingredient in all of my treatment. I have a sign on my bathroom mirror, reminding me.

I am now in drug treatment. The first chemo drug erased the tumors on the pleura. Now the breast cancer (ER+) has metastasized to my liver and that requires another drug. The side effects are crazy. At least I can stay home through this treatment period.

Recently I tried medical marijuana for the abdominal pain associated with the drug Xeloda. I was pleasantly surprised to feel the pain subside but was not happy to be smoking again, even though it isn't tobacco.

I learned the process of getting an Arizona Medical Marijuana card and will try another form such as oil or a capsule. The process began with collecting a year's worth of medical documentation and making an appointment at the Natural Healing Center to see one of their doctors.

At the appointment the doctor looked at my medical records and we discussed my symptoms to determine my eligibility. The doctor decided I was eligible and signed the necessary documents. My application for a Medical Marijuana Card was submitted to the State. These papers were all sent to the Arizona Department of Health Services. It was easier than I imagined.

I am thankful that I had a teaching career. Helping children learn and seeing the "aha" in their eyes is most rewarding. Through the school system I have a pension and enough income to meet my expenses.

Thank you, God!

KEN

PROSTATE
CANCER

Age 68
when diagnosed

KEN – PROSTATE CANCER

Ken served in the U.S. Army, and did two tours of duty in The Republic of Viet Nam where "Agent Orange" chemicals were used. As a result of Agent Orange many men were diagnosed with prostate cancer at some point following their service. Ken began Prostate Specific Antigen (PSA) tests on an annual basis beginning in 1980.

In addition, his primary care physician began digital rectal exams, checking out the gland that normally is the size of a walnut. In 2012 Ken's PSA scores began climbing.

A biopsy of the prostate gland was ordered and blood work was done. A Gleason Score (in a range of 1-5) is used as a measure to detect cancer. Ken's score was low and the biopsy score was 2-3. He was told to wait six months. Worry worked on his mind and Ken began his own research about cancer of the prostate. WebMD, Mayo Clinic and American Cancer Society are credible sources.

By 2014 two more biopsies had been performed and the Gleason Score was now elevated to the 4-5 range. Ken's initial reaction was "let's tackle it." By now he was seeing his urologist, a radiologist and a surgeon. This was confusing and caused a dilemma. Ken had to make choices that could impact him the rest of his life.

1) The radiologist explained that radiation kills everything in order to stop the spread of cancer. It may involve the placement of pellets that would then be radiated, based on areas where the biopsy showed cancerous tissue.

2) The surgeon's plan was "preferred surgery." He would remove the whole gland. Body function could change to incontinence (loss of bladder control) and inability to maintain an erection. *If the cancer was confined in the prostate gland Ken would be considered cancer free.*

3) A third option was "watchful waiting" and that caused anxiety.

Following more research Ken decided to consult a different surgeon who was recommended by friends. Dr. Sanjay Ramakumar, MD, of Arizona Institute of Urology, explained the surgery he performs most often (at least 600).

In an hour and a half meeting with Ken and his wife Gail he explained the benefit of the "DaVinci" surgery. It is considered a robotic procedure because the doctor can see and magnify the tunnel to the gland. He manipulates metal arms and hands to move a tendon or a nerve, enlarge the working area, and get a better view inside the body in three-dimension. This method preserves as much function as possible. The patient experiences less blood loss and minimal pain. Details and videos of the "DaVinci" can be found online at "davincisurgery.com."

After hearing all the details Ken felt satisfied that this was the right choice for him. Confident that he now had the right surgeon and the right method for eliminating the prostate cancer,

Ken checked into the hospital on December 14, 2014 with surgery scheduled for the next day. Shortly after surgery he was able to stand and walk around the bed. The next day he walked further. There was little pain and he went home on Dec. 16 with a colostomy bag and catheter, but no prostate gland.

After surgery a physical therapist showed him urinary exercises to do three times a day and said that soon he would return to normal function. The catheter and colostomy were removed ten days after surgery. Later, Viagra provided a satisfying sexual performance.

Ken was surprised when he was told there were still some margin cells and he would have a blood draw every three months. At this time his PSA numbers are in the range of 0.01 and 0.02.

Quality of life is important to Ken and his wife. She has partnered with him throughout the ordeal. They have attended several support group meetings and have benefitted from the speakers and hearing of each other's experience with prostate cancer.

Ken believes that physical therapy is critical to recovery. His urologist is thorough and supportive. Ken is not limited in activities and plans are being made for travel.

++

GAIL – WIFE AND HELPMATE

Ken and Gail have been married since 1994. Gail was frustrated with the process of finding doctors and being unable to sit down with all of them for consultation. Ken's primary care doctor helped pull it all together and his recommendations helped. Ken spent a long time researching the various options and remained upbeat; never depressed.

Ken was healthy prior to the day he was given a diagnosis of cancer. Yet, he approached the whole scenario as a project that required him to learn as much as possible before making any commitments.

"Ken takes good care of himself and enjoys my cooking," says Gail. They have worked together to create a healthy diet. Gail mentions that their sex life is satisfying since the surgery. She is very happy with Ken's decisions and felt he had excellent care and a quick recovery.

Ken likes to golf and Gail teaches yoga.

MIRIAM

CANCER OF
THE TONGUE

Age 74
when diagnosed

MIRIAM – CANCER OF THE TONGUE

December 2014 – Our Christmas newsletter

"A Merry Christmas and a blessed New Year is our prayer for you. May the Love of this season enfold you and strengthen you.

Our daily lives seem ho-hum and routine. However, some things have changed. Because of Chuck's Alzheimer's, he hasn't golfed in over a year. I too am not golfing and I've cut down on my Bridge games in order to be home with him. Chuck has trouble finding and forming the right words so socializing is difficult. However, he is still loving and caring and interested in others. Our life is what it is--and right now it is still good."

Chuck and Miriam

Their two adult children, Chuck and Cindi, their spouses and children, live in the northeastern part of the United States.

Miriam's story is taken from her emails and those of her children, as indicated by parentheses.

January 13, 2015 (Miriam)

Before Christmas, Chuck and I each had an appointment with our dermatologist. She found a "suspicious" spot on Chuck's right back shoulder and did a biopsy. It is melanoma and today she did the surgery and removed a golf ball diameter hunk. All was removed and she didn't think it necessary for him to receive any further treatment.

She looked at sores on my tongue and cheeks and said follow-up would be needed. Today, I got "numbed up" and a slice was taken off my tongue to be sent for biopsy. I have lost 60 pounds because there is tongue pain when I try to eat. Speaking also causes pain. I have been diagnosed with cancer of the tongue.

Son Chuck flew in to Tennessee on Sunday, to accompany me to the oncologist appointment and will head back to Connecticut this afternoon. It is so good to have him here to talk things over. He spent several hours sorting through our large LP record collection--making three piles--1) donate, 2) review, and 3) keep. The review pile will keep me busy for several days.

February 11 (Miriam)

I met once again with my oncologist. He has formulated what drugs I will be taking. The plan is chemo once a week for three weeks, then a week off. This will last about four months. Now the insurance company has to look it over and give approval. That could take two weeks. "Sigh."

 I am ready to get started. The doctor checked the port he installed and said it is doing very well. I will meet with the radiation doctor again to get things rolling.

February 19 (Miriam)

The phone call came today. My first chemo will be the morning of February 26th. It's starting.

February 24 (Miriam)

Early last week we had an ice storm; then, another big storm with sleet, ice pellets, and high winds. Much of our area is without electricity and heat. Neighbors have been in and out. Chuck is bored with no TV and no computer for his games.

February 26 (Miriam)

Son Chuck drove from Connecticut to go with me to my first chemo this morning. Port was flushed, blood was tested, and I was given an IV of Benadryl and anti-nausea medicine.

My oncologist came in and chatted, asking when my radiation was scheduled. I told him March 9. Everything stopped! Chemo and radiation are supposed to be done at the same time.

I'm bummed out. Son Chuck will leave in the morning, driving back to CT. Big disappointment. "Take a big breath and get on with it," I tell myself.

March 9 (Miriam)

Daughter Cindi came in from Washington D.C. to be with me for chemo and radiation. Today was a BIG day, but I don't feel any different. I'm so thankful for the cards and prayers.

When I go to the radiation treatment I lie on a bed. The technicians put a previously fitted solid mesh mask on my face. Then a popsicle-like device is put through an opening in the mask and into my mouth. I am told to bite lightly on it. This is to keep my head from moving during the treatment. The mask is very snug, but not uncomfortable.

Friends and neighbors have supported us, providing rides for me as needed and keeping Dad, Chuck from getting into trouble.

March 18 (Miriam)

I've had two chemo treatments and one and a half weeks of radiation. No side effects yet. Doctors want me to GAIN weight--a first in my life. I have trouble chewing and nothing tastes good. Cindi was here for the first week. She took me to my appointments, did shopping and cooking, and entertained her dad, along with other tasks.

Cindi left Saturday and son Chuck flew in on Sunday. His job allows him to work anywhere and he will be here a couple of weeks. He intended to be with me for chemo and radiation but for now I can drive myself, leaving him time to spend with his Dad.

March 22 (Miriam)

For two days I have been very sleepy--can "drop off" any time I close my eyes. I awaken with a sore throat. My lips are swollen and chapped. I can't bear to think of eating or drinking anything. I've lost ten pounds this week. Tomorrow I will get IV fluids.

March 25 (Miriam)

Today I was going to drive myself to treatments, but my eyesight was "off." So son Chuck and Dad drove me. Then I discovered that I was wearing Dad's glasses!

April 1 (Son Chuck)

Mom was admitted to the hospital today. Her blood pressure was low and she had noticeably lost strength and was having trouble walking. She is halfway through radiation and one quarter of the way through chemotherapy. She is not taking anything by mouth and is not talking. She had a feeding tube surgically inserted. No visitors please.

The situation at home has been complex with Dad not remembering or understanding that Mom is sick. We are pursuing moving him to an assisted living home near here.

April 4 (Son Chuck)

Mom came home today and is getting around with a walker. We have done several feedings through the tube.

I read 6 pages of email to her and she smiled with her cheeks and eyes. She sleeps most of the time. Dad's love for my mother is apparent even though he did not notice Mom's absence or return.

April 9 (Cindi)

Mom had both chemo and radiation today, is feeling stronger and gaining weight. Yesterday was pretty tough. We moved Dad to a nearby assisted care place. He was confused and did not understand what was happening.

Today my brother and husband visited him in the morning. A friend took him out to lunch and I visited in the evening. He is in great spirits--has stated that he likes the place and the people.

He had no trouble saying good-bye. I keep reminding myself-- baby steps. It will take some getting used to for all of us. Thank you for the supportive messages and your prayers. They are working!

April 11 (Cindi)

I took the kids over to play a little baseball with Dad. What a hoot for all of us!

April 15 (Cindi)

Our goal now is independence. Mom is learning to use the feeding tube to deliver her meds and liquid food. She walks without the walker and is gaining weight.

Keeping track of her blood sugar is a challenge. We still need to find a good way for her to wake up when it is time to "eat" and take her meds. The pain medication is adequate but makes her tired. If she doesn't get up then her blood sugar will be too low and she will be really confused about what to do. With hearing loss she doesn't hear the phone or the alarm.

April 17 (Cindi)

I will stay with Mom until my brother arrives. A visiting nurse will come on Monday to assess physical needs as well as help with transportation.

Dad seems happy when we visit, but has been packing his suitcase with all of his things every day. A few nights ago, he walked out with his suitcase into the rain and was persuaded by the staff to return. He doesn't really grasp what is happening.

This home is not a lock down facility, so, this afternoon we visited Victorian Square 40 miles away. It is what it is--a nursing home with a memory care unit--which may be what Dad needs.

We will continue to look at options. Please keep visiting him. He loves to chat and sing, walk around the grounds and go get ice cream. He is still good natured and perks up from interaction with others.

May 14 (Miriam)

I just had a chemo treatment where all went fine! Then I had a short consult with the radiation doctor. I did my feeding and will now sit and put my feet up for a while.

May 19 (Miriam)

Life is good here. There are a few "hiccups" occasionally, but day by day I'm feeling better. Chemo continues for another month or so.

THE STORY OF A SURVIVOR
See cover photo

I was looking in my back yard the other day and saw the peony plants blooming with delicate pink flowers. Chuck's parents lived in Dearborn MI and had a garden of vegetables and flowers. When his dad died we sold the house.

I took one of the peony plants and transplanted it in our Dearborn yard. It bloomed regularly for 20 years. Then we moved to TN. The peony was one of the plants that survived the move. It was plopped into the ground and got no extra attention.

Now, another 20 years later it is still blooming-- spreading its joy and hope. It's not a prize winner, but it certainly is a survivor!!

Bloom where planted is something to be remembered. Spread beauty and hope. God is good.

June 5 (Miriam)

When the radiation finished a couple of weeks ago, I thought things would get easier. I guess they have, but other issues have to be dealt with. I am not able to talk or swallow and cannot use the phone. I am told to give it time and then work with a therapist.

The radiation left me with a very bad sunburn-like condition on my neck and upper chest. It is now healing and only two spots are still tender. I have reflux that makes socializing and sleeping difficult. No one wants to listen to me gagging and spitting up. However, it is getting better.

Then there is my feeding tube. It had been working well, but lately started leaking and finally became detached. So, I went to the hospital and was anesthetized while a replacement feeding tube was placed into my stomach. After a consult with the oncologist, I had a two unit blood transfusion.

Meanwhile Cindi came and took charge of moving her dad to an Alzheimer's facility 40 miles from our home. She had so many decisions to make with little time and no help from me. She is amazing.

Through all of this, I've discovered a few things:

❖ My sense of humor is still here, but most of the time it is deeply buried.

❖ I am much more self-centered and selfish than I thought I could ever be. I know that at this time it is okay, but it is still quite startling.

❖ I knew I would have prayers and support and help from friends, but it has been overwhelming. So many have offered their help. Cards come almost daily. Emails continue to strengthen and support me. I have been blessed daily as friends assure me they are praying for me every step of the way.

❖ Losing my husband to Alzheimer's has made a double burden for our children as they grieve for the Dad they knew and loved. He is physically there, but this disease is cruel because there is no recognition of family members and friends. Chuck embodied the meaning of love. He was a good golfer, a beautiful singer, a caring and gentle Christian man.

June 12 (Miriam)

This week went well. Yesterday my blood work was excellent, so I had chemo – only two more to go.

I have two gripes:

Gripe #1

I still have a rather severe radiation burn on my neck, shoulders, and upper chest. At a meeting with the radiation nurses, I was told to use Aloe. I bought some and used it. The next week they said use Aquaphor. I bought some and used it. The next week they said use Eucerin. I bought some and used it. Cocoa butter was also suggested. None of them helped. Finally I was given a prescription for Silvadene and that began the healing I desperately needed.

Gripe #2

Many medical people are telling me that I should be swallowing water and talking by now. Yesterday two nurses lectured me about how I should be swallowing and talking. <u>Then</u>, they looked in my mouth and were shocked at the amount of sores on my tongue and remarked how painful it must be. Well yeah. Duh! Things are improving but not as quickly as we all want.

I love to read and figured with time on my hands I would spend it reading. However, my limited concentration doesn't allow it. What a disappointment.

I get stronger each day. I do all of the household chores and have even pruned the bushes! Friend Naiad and Cindi bought clothes for me--I was still wearing my very big shirts and slacks. Now I can go out in public and "strut" my 147 pound self.

June 17 (Miriam)

My life isn't just about cancer. My dryer stopped heating at the age of 20 years so I decided to replace it. On Lowe's website I found one with features I want and ordered it. Then, my next door neighbor pulled my dryer out and looked at it. He found it was plugged into a 110 volt rather than a 220. Today an electrician came out and told me what needed to be done.

I have a clothesline in the garage and neighbors have offered use of their dryers. It still amazes me that friends jump in whatever the need. I am truly blessed.

June 20 (Miriam)

The feeding tube is leaking and so I basically have had no calories or nourishment for the last two days. I am on my way to the hospital where blood work is good. Diabetes reading is fine. Two chest x-rays, one stomach x-ray, and IV saline for dehydration.

A doctor came and looked at the feeding tube. It is no longer in the stomach. Nothing will go
into my body for the next 36 hours. My friend Sue, again, was a real trooper. She asked the right questions, held my hand and in that I found comfort!

June 22 (Miriam)

My feeding at home did not go well. Once again the substance did not go into my stomach. So, it was back to the hospital where I stayed ten long days. The tube is secure and I am able to feed myself. My weight is 138. I don't remember ever being that weight.

Yesterday I had an appointment with the oncologist, who said I didn't need the last chemo. Yeah! He has set a PET Scan for July 9. Once again I needed and had help from local friends. I am so blessed.

My new dryer has been installed and performs admirably. One more thing I can take off my list.

HAPPY BIRTHDAY!

to my grandson Weller and Son Chuck.

I'm upset that so many special occasions have slipped by.

July 6 (Miriam)

I have finished radiation and chemo. I feel stronger daily. Son Chuck is flying in to go with me to the doctor as scheduled next Monday.

When the mail came today there were several cards of support. I started thinking about all these past months where EVERY DAY there have been one or more greeting cards in the mail. It has been overwhelming. Some of you sent many, some several, and some just one. They have all touched me.

Please know that I have felt your love, caring and support. We're not done yet, so keep the prayers coming. God bless you all.

July 9 (Miriam)

My PET scan was early and all went smoothly. Then I went to a surgery follow-up appointment. The doctor looked at the sites and liked what he saw. He removed my stitches. I came home, had a feeding, and now am going to work on a jigsaw puzzle.

July 13 (Miriam)

Saw the oncologist today to discuss results of last week's PET scan, and I quote; "The areas of abnormal activity in the left mandible is absent on this study. Small amounts of activity in the maxilla may be related to periodontal changes. Overall improvement."

There will be no more radiation, nor chemo. Next step is to see the ear, nose and throat doctor. He will look at the report, schedule an endoscopy and biopsy. Day by day I am stronger and have more energy.

July 16 (Miriam)

The ear, nose, and throat doctor saw NO suspicious sites! However, the tongue is still in bad shape from radiation necrosis and sloughing. He also saw fungus/bacteria that will probably take four to six months of healing. I now have several different mouth washes to use frequently and regularly. He saw NO reason for a biopsy. Good news.

July 18 (Cindi)

First, some background information about Dad. When he was at Fairfield Glade Assisted Living, which is not a memory facility, he often asked the ladies, "How about a kiss?" If they said no, he walked away. If they said yes, he would peck on the cheek. This was not seen as inappropriate behavior in that setting.

Since he moved to Clarity Pointe this routine continued. However, ladies he is addressing cannot answer him or do not really understand. Residents were getting upset and husbands of residents were also bothered, seeing it as inappropriate. The nurse changed his mood-altering drugs and has been making changes for a while, trying to find the right balance.

This week, whether because of the meds, or because of the degenerative nature of Alzheimer's, or some combination of both, Dad became very agitated, combative, hostile and violent. On Wednesday he was waving his putter at people and pushed a staff member against the wall. He is angry but not able to communicate why.

The staff was able to sedate him and a pastor friend came and sat with him for awhile. The next day was not good and finally yesterday afternoon, they made a call to have him transported to a hospital emergency room because he was a danger to the staff and residents.

Since there was no "psych" bed available at the time, he was sedated and put in restraints. The hope was that he would be admitted for a 48 hour observation and they could work on his meds.

I spoke with someone from ER just now. Dad is out of the restraints, but still very agitated. They are trying to get him calm enough so he can be transported to a Psych unit at another hospital. They will accept him only if he is <u>not</u> combative!

July 19 (Cindi)

I have been in contact with Park West Hospital a few times throughout the day. Dad has been admitted to critical care. He will be staying there with no plans to transfer to another facility for right now.

He had an MRI and a CT scan today, and tomorrow I will hear from the doctor about the results of those tests. Dad has had visits from the psych doctors who have come to his room since there are no psych bed openings right now. I believe he is in good hands.

July 22 (Cindi)

Managing my dad's care from so far away is a challenge. After jumping through <u>many</u> hoops to get information, I learned that Dad is still in critical care. He has not been eating and is periodically in restraints. He is disoriented and agitated. He pulled out his IV and tried to leave. It is hard for me to be at home so far away, but I was assured a visit now is not wise.

July 25 (Cindi)

I had quite a scare today. I called Park West Hospital for an update and was told Dad had been discharged. Where? Not Clarity Pointe. Finally I learned he was admitted to the Senior Behavior Program at Park West. They needed to do a new admission and kept calling Mom. She doesn't answer the phone since she cannot talk. It knocked the wind out of me.

Since Dad was moved to Senior Behavior he has been confused, agitated, and combative. Security got involved a few times, which sounds scary but makes sense because he is not on any psych meds.

July 27 (Cindi)

Dad has improved. He is out of restraints, eating, and taking a low dose of anxiety meds. I

I know there is no cure for Alzheimer's but today's conversations gave me hope that he will go back to Clarity Pointe sometime soon.

July 31 – (Miriam)

I'm talking now – words, not paragraphs, so phone calls don't work. Last week I went to the local theater, played bridge and am going to a memorial service at church tomorrow. I'm starting to have a life again.

August 2 – (Miriam)

Cindi got a call from the hospital that her dad, who was admitted two weeks ago for Alzheimer's related aggression, is now in acute kidney failure. He is not producing any urine – even with an IV and a catheter. They want to know how we feel about continuing medical help or should they just keep him comfortable.

In a conference call with Cindi and my pastor, we gave permission to have a nephrologist (kidney specialist) do some tests in the morning so we would have more information on which to base our decision.

August 4 (Cindi)

Well, the results of the CT scan showed that there was no obstruction with his kidneys. It is a true case of kidney failure. The nurse today told me that as of last night, Dad could no longer swallow his food. He is becoming unaware of his body.

Mom made the decision to end treatment and he will be receiving comfort care—pain meds only. They will begin this at the hospital, but may move him to a hospice, depending on how long he holds on. Mom had a friend take her to the hospital this afternoon to see him. Please keep them in your prayers.

August 4 (Cindi)

I was telling my sons why I was going to Tennessee tomorrow (to say good-bye to my dad) and I was crying. Charlie, my six year old said, "Why is everyone crying if he is going to heaven?" Charlie knows that I am not sure what I believe, but he is very clear on what he believes.

August 6 – (Miriam)

Both my son and daughter arrived last night within an hour of each other. Dad is being transported to Hospice in a nearby city. His belongings will be packed and moved back home from Clarity Pointe.

The family is gathering. Meanwhile, I nap and feed myself like the "princess" I sometimes pretend to be. Ha! Cindi had planned to drive to Dearborn, MI for a high school reunion and son Chuck and I encouraged her to go. She already said goodbye to her dad.

August 7 (Miriam)

Son Chuck and I got a phone call from Hospice telling us that it would be good if we could come. We did and sat with my husband Chuck for about 45 minutes before he died. He is in a far, far better place. Thanks to all of you for being with us – in person and in your thoughts and prayers.

A friend asked how I was coping and my reply was that my husband began leaving me in 2008 when he was diagnosed with Alzheimer's disease. He has been outside our home for the past six months. I guess I've been grieving for a long time. Now I rest, knowing that Chuck is in Heaven with a body that knows no illness.

August 15 (Miriam)

A Memorial service was held at our church, Christ Lutheran, where, over the years, Chuck served as Treasurer and President of Council He was active in barbershop music for many years.

Chuck was an active participant of Via de Cristo in both Michigan and Tennessee. He woke each day with a sense of gratitude, and lived a good life. He and I were married 52 years.

August 17 (Miriam)

A good friend is staying with me for a week. We have dealt with death certificates, Social Security, the bank, and life insurance. We also went shopping for new clothes--size 10.

September 2 (Miriam)

This afternoon I had a follow-up appointment with my radiologist. He gave me a thorough examination and then told me he had read all the reports and sees no cancer.

My tongue is still swollen and there are still sores in my mouth. I can't swallow anything. The doctor told me to be patient. It may be a month or more before there is significant improvement.

September 3 (Miriam)

Well, I took another step toward being normal. The visiting nurse agreed with me that I am ready to be discharged. That means I can now drive myself wherever I want to go.

I so appreciate all of the help I had getting to appointments and other places, but I am really excited about doing it myself as I did before. My hair is growing in quickly and no, it is not coming in curly.

September 13 (Miriam)

My calendar is full with fun activities. I have been weeding an hour at a time. My concentration is much better and I can read again.

September 19 (Miriam)

We have planned the committal service for Chuck's cremains at the Columbarium at Christ Lutheran Church. I am adjusting to my new life and I thank God for many things.

October 2 (Miriam)

The weather has turned cool so I shopped for sweaters, long sleeved tops, winter coat and a windbreaker.

I saw my primary care physician who checked me over, ordered blood-work and gave me a shot for poison ivy that I didn't see when working in the yard. My mouth is still "uncomfortable" but much better than it was.

Several days ago I read a paragraph in "The Upper Room" devotional book that said what has been in my heart. I paraphrased, inserting my name.

"Today, we give thanks to God for Miriam. She has endured great trials--but not alone. Many people have helped, encouraging her with prayers, and timely assistance. Miriam now smiles with happiness and confidence. God, her constant companion, worked a miracle of love and healing. God was and is a very real presence in Miriam's life."

October 12 (Miriam)

This past week was quite interesting. I scheduled a hearing exam and it showed my left ear was somewhat damaged from the radiation, but my hearing aid could be tweaked. The doctor told me she sold her practice and will retire at the age of 50.

Then I went for my yearly exam by my dermatologist. She is no longer doing exams, only surgeries. At least I had a few moments with her to thank her for diagnosing my tongue cancer. I was introduced to the new doctor and passed the exam.

Next I stopped at the eye doctor's office where Chuck and I were regular patients. There was only one car in the parking lot. My ophthalmologist retired two weeks ago. The woman who fit eye glasses in an adjoining office died a year ago.

It is hard to believe that four of my health professionals have changed for one reason or another. All this happened in the year of my cancer.

To make the day feel better I stopped to look at new cars and decided on a 2016 Ford Escape. I had two vehicles to trade.

As if that wasn't enough, I saw the oncologist and he said, "You are cancer free." He ordered a PET scan with follow-up on October 23rd. He also wrote an order for me to start swallowing therapy. I am ready. I am grateful that I have the emotional and physical strength to handle these things.

October 23 (Miriam)

Fall is here and it is warm. The beautiful leaves are falling too quickly--I need more time to look at them. I have managed to keep up with the necessary raking. Thank you over and over for the support and love you, my friends and family, have shown. My love to you all, Miriam

Mid-January, 2016 (Miriam)

My tongue is still swollen, but not nearly as big as it was. I have been talking for a couple of months now but only for a short time. It doesn't take long for my throat to begin hurting. If I sing I start "squeaking." I am learning "patience!!"

I just returned from my appointment with the swallowing therapist. I was able to take in and swallow some banana baby food and some thickened nectar. This will not be for nutrition, rather to exercise the area and get used to the swallowing procedure again--something I never thought about before.

Last week I saw radiology videos of my swallowing and it still shows considerable swelling in the area, but everything is working. I thank God for the medical expertise available and for your continued prayers.

I am blessed.

May 3, 2016 (Miriam)

In the past week I saw a specialist, who after discussion, was going to arrange for me to have a larger diameter feeding tube put into my stomach to minimize the leaking I was experiencing.

Well, would you believe that now the leaking is almost non-existent? I haven't done anything differently, so what is happening?

Then I had my "AHA" moment. After I sent out my message, many of you started praying intentionally...knowing what to pray for. And it worked!! I am not surprised, but why am I surprised? HA.

I phoned the specialist this afternoon and cancelled the procedure and was assured that I could start it up again if needed.

Other good news: I started "eating" this past week. I had Jello Chocolate/Vanilla pudding two afternoons in a row and all went well.

The next day I had Jello Strawberry Cheesecake pudding and it went down easily also. However, that evening when I tested my blood sugar it was really high. Scary high. I "treated" myself with insulin and by morning was back to normal.

I haven't "eaten" anything since. I will be making an appointment with a nutritionist to guide me through this next step--what to eat, whether to cut down on the tube feedings, etc.

So this is a good news memo. May 1 was the year anniversary of my last radiation treatment and I can look back and see the giant strides that have been made. Still a ways to go, but it feels like it will be mostly "downhill" and quicker and easier now.

Thank you all and may God continue to bless us. Miriam.

May 22, 2016

Today was a BIG day for me.

First a little history lesson:

When I was a child our church had Holy Communion only 4 times a year and you had to announce your intention to take Communion the week prior. It was all very special and awe-filled. When I finished my confirmation classes and could partake of this Sacrament, I was filled with such JOY.

Now we celebrate this Sacrament weekly and I know the reasons for the change and agree with them, but I also sometimes miss the reverence that we used to experience.

Because of my health issues, I have not taken Communion for over a year. I know that I am still loved completely and that my Salvation is assured because of Him. However, there has been this void.

Today I was able to go up to the Table and Eat and Drink. I was overcome with that old sense of awe and reverence and thankfulness. Almost like that first time 62 years ago.

 Praise the Lord!

The hymn on the next page gave me great comfort throughout my treatment.

Healer of Our Every Ill

"(Refrain) Healer of our every ill, light of each tomorrow, give us peace beyond our fear and hope beyond our sorrow.

You, who know our fears and sadness, grace us with your peace and gladness. Spirit of all comfort, fill our hearts.

In the pain and joy, beholding how your grace is still unfolding, give us all your vision, God of love.

Give us strength to love each other, every sister, every brother. Spirit of all kindness, be our guide.

You who know each thought and feeling, teach us all your way of healing. Spirit of compassion, fill each heart."

MARGARET

BREAST
CANCER

Age 46
when diagnosed

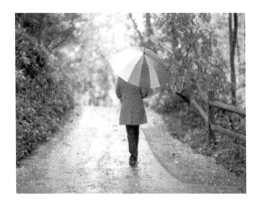

Each of us walks the path of the unknown on a daily basis. Events occur that we could neither predict nor plan for. A phone call informed us this morning that my step-daughter was in an accident that totaled her car. She was on her way home from work. Extent of injuries is still unknown.

In walking this path, I look toward the light that to me represents the guidance, comfort and support of the Holy Spirit.

MARGARET PHALOR SCHROF BARNHART
BREAST CANCER

January, 1987

I felt the lump in my breast as I showered one Friday evening. In that moment the expectation of having fun at a friend's birthday party diminished.

Should I call the doctor Monday? Surely I'm over-reacting. If I wait several weeks it may go away. Socializing at the celebration was hampered by three trips to the bathroom to feel the lump that was still there.

After a mammogram and a course of antibiotics for a possible milk gland infection, the lump was still there and I was referred to a surgeon. He pressed on my breast and found two more lumps and did a needle biopsy on all three palpable lumps. He called to tell me that one lump appeared to be cancerous.

At the age of 46 this information was overpowering and I tucked it to the back of my mind as I headed to my graduate class in art therapy. It was impossible not to think about it but I didn't say anything to fellow students.

During my appointment with the surgeon he told me I would need a mastectomy. I questioned why not a lumpectomy as I had recently read about. His response was that the mastectomy has been done since the 1800's and was the best treatment. Huh? But this is 1987!

I wanted a second opinion and asked a number of people who they would recommend. Going to a larger city and speaking with another surgeon, I was given good reasons to have a mastectomy. He based his opinion on the size of the lump, the size of my breast, and the location of the tumor.

Now I understood the whole picture, and was ready to sign consent for my small town surgeon to do a mastectomy. But first, I had to decide what to do about "Handicap Awareness Days." I had organized a day at both of my elementary schools, involving all students in Grades 1-5. It involved stations set up in the gym and parent volunteers. The week prior I had gone into the classrooms to prepare the students for what they would experience. My decision was to go ahead with it.

Following the mastectomy I was amused when remembering that one of the activities for the kids required them to perform various tasks with one hand tied behind their back. Following the surgery I was forced to use my left hand when I was dominant on the right.

The doctors were concerned that so much time passed before the surgery, but it was important to me to grasp and to understand what I would experience and to feel ready. Today, the surgeons generally agree it is not necessary to rush this decision.

I knew very little about breast cancer and at the age of 46 no one among my family or friends had dealt with it. The difference between then and now is huge. Today the pink ribbons are prominent and those diagnosed feel free to tell their story on television, in books and in movies.

Cancer centers and support groups provide guidance for the patient. Much has changed since 1987. With internet access a woman can gain a great deal of information that she can talk over with medical personnel. Some men are diagnosed with breast cancer and the internet can offer support to them as well as women.

A mastectomy is a process where the surgeon makes an incision and scoops the tissue out of the breast. (I thought they amputated it.) The doctor will preserve the nipple if possible. Nerves and muscles are retained to the greatest extent. Normally the doctor will remove one or more lymph nodes from the arm- pit so they can be evaluated and determined if cancer is present there. If so, there is a possibility that the cancer has spread to other parts of the body. The incision is closed and drainage tubes are placed.

If the woman has chosen reconstruction, a plastic surgeon will be present to initiate the process before the incision is closed. A number of options are available and the patient is advised to look into the possibilities. In my case I was advised not to have reconstruction for at least a year. The surgeon wanted clear x-rays of the breast area. At the end of the year, I decided against reconstruction for three reasons--the pain involved, lack of nerve sensation in the nipple, and I was well adjusted to my prosthesis.

March

The discovery of the tumor, the mastectomy, the diagnosis of cancer and the beginning of chemotherapy, all began with an emotional shock.

The grief cycle had begun--not once, but four times, over the course of a month. First was feeling the lump; second the biopsy results; third the mastectomy; and fourth, chemotherapy.

I experienced the full range of emotions through each grief cycle until resolution was reached. It took a long time. My tumbling thoughts and feelings were like being the ball in a game of handball, not knowing which way the ball will be coming.

A grief cycle is not lineal. It bounces around and some feelings hang on for a very long time and others appear, disappear and then return. Shock is usually first in the cycle. There will also be disbelief, confusion, bargaining, and anger (often experienced as depression) and a whole range of feelings stacked unevenly on top of each other.

Depression was probably the hardest for me and it lasted a long time. Faith and religious beliefs were searched. People diagnosed with life-threatening illness often ask "Why me?" while I thought "Why not me?" I had a support team, nearby facilities, and super insurance benefits.

Different friends had different skills, knowledge and demeanor and I would ask the person I needed, at any one time, to help. Years later, changes in my personal life, professional counseling and anti-depressant medications brought me out of depression.

I didn't talk to anyone about the over-powering feelings. Instead I reached the depth of my soul and expressed myself in writing free-style poetry and drawing--usually around 2:00 am when I couldn't sleep.

My parents were my model and I kept most of the emotional turmoil to myself. When my dad was diagnosed with Hodgkin's disease in his 30's the doctor told <u>him</u> that he had cancer and the outcome, though unknown, did not look good.

The doctor met with my mother and told her to prepare for my dad's death. I was eight years old and felt the tension even though I didn't know the cause.

The best known treatment at that time was radiation, used to kill the cancer cells. It worked and Dad lived a full life. Cancer came back in the form of Lymphoma when he was in his 70's.

The last time I saw him was in a hospital bed with tubes going in and coming out. He had been on chemo for a year but it was no longer strong enough to eliminate the cancer.

My dad and I had a casual conversation and he died several days later. I will always regret that he and I didn't talk about his impending death. Perhaps it was too difficult for both of us.

It wasn't until my diagnosis of cancer that my mother told me the story of what happened when I was eight years old. The message I heard that day was, "Don't talk about it."

What follows includes some of the free-style poetry written during my cancer event in 1987. It focuses on chemotherapy.

[The words in italics are from "Journey Unknown, 2nd Edition, 2012, Focusing on the Emotional Aspect of Cancer, Mastectomy and Chemotherapy]

(THE PARADOX)

Cancer is a life-threatening disease.
People die of cancer—
        many women, many men.
Having cancer does not mean
I will die of cancer.

April   (THE CHEMOTHERAPY CRISIS)

'Good news,' said the surgeon.
'Lymph nodes are clear, we got it all.'

'Not so good,' says my internist, as he explains that for my type of cancer I need at least six months of chemotherapy.

But I hate to experience nausea, and I don't want to lose my hair.

My father endured the treatment for a year before he died.

I fear the chemicals. Do I also fear the possibility of death?

My son and I were working a puzzle on the dining room table the evening before my first infusion of chemotherapy drugs. He was a senior in high school. I told him I didn't intend to die of cancer.

He told me I would probably get hit by a car on the way to my last IV! Through my tears, I laughed.

Upon arriving home, I anticipated nausea and vomiting, along with weakness, so I took a bucket into the bedroom with me and lay down on the bed, and covered myself with a quilt. I waited-- for an hour. Nothing happened. I waited for another hour. Nothing happened. So I got up, put the bucket away, and began to fix dinner.

April (FEAR AND TEARS)

Listen to me doctor, understand my tears.
The pain of losing a breast has dimmed.

Fear of chemotherapy and unknown side- effects immobilizes me.
Pills to take and the first IV.

Halfway through the night I sit--afraid to fall asleep.
I want to stay awake, so I know I am alive.

Three weeks of chemo and I was experiencing fatigue. My husband informed me there was an ice-skating show in town and we decided to go.

Into the shower and a quick shampoo brought me to my knees. I had a hand full of hair. I expected it, but not all at once. I had a wad of hair. It was stunning disbelief and simultaneous knowledge that I am not to be spared this side-effect. Tears poured down my cheeks as we sat in the darkness of the ice-skating show.

I lived in small town Ohio with my husband and a son who was a senior in high school. Our oldest son lived in a distant city. Prior to the mastectomy I worked as an elementary school counselor in a larger city thirty miles away.

Although I drove myself to the doctor's office to get my IV's, I was unable to drive to my school. Even if I arrived safely the side- effects of chemo, especially weakness and poor concentration, prohibited me from working.

No-one I knew had experienced mastectomy or chemotherapy (other than my father.) Taking this journey was frightening and lonely. My hair was mostly gone and became the first public sign of my treatment. When I went shopping for a wig, I selected one similar to my natural hair color. I didn't know you could get it washed, cut and styled, so it never looked quite right. Without it my head was cold and with it my head was hot. Options for head covering were almost non-existent, in 1987.

May   (THREE REFLECTIONS)

I look in the mirror. Who am I?
In the reflection I see a curly-headed blond.
Out into the world I go, feeling the wig covering my head, wondering who notices. I was feigning confidence, trying to forget.

I look in the mirror. Who am I now? In the reflection I see a thin-haired old woman.
Telling others it's like a baby's fine hair, trying to deny the real thoughts, the old woman thoughts.

I look in the mirror. Who am I now?
In the reflection, I see a cover-up.

Feeling my head getting cold in the comfort of my home, I add a scarf that offers warmth and hides reality.

A scarf--and yet another symbol that I have cancer.

May   (LIVING FOR TODAY)

I've quit fighting--because I've given up?--given in?

*No.   It's more like giving over, giving way.
Too much is outside my control.*

I'll accept what is. I'll live for today.

*I cannot add one day to my life.
I'll do what I can for the moment.*

May   (CONTROL)

I've lost control. I flounder.

Yet, I sense an inward flow from a spiritual source that goes through me and radiates out to others, deepening in meaning as it travels, continuing in its movement back to me and giving meaning to my life.

But, what do I control?

Unexpected happenings cause change: physical, emotional, mental, spiritual, and social.

What controls me? (Or, Who controls me?)

Notice the difference between the first line and the last. When I say "I've lost control" it is self-centered and expresses my thought that I actually had control of my life.

However, cancer taught me that it is not within my power to control much of what was happening. I could make choices regarding my treatment and choice of doctors, or I could refuse treatment.

I often thought about the possibility of dying instead of going into remission. I asked God to talk to me but I wasn't a very good listener. I neglected to look for and feel His comfort.

My Christian beliefs were buried somewhere within me, but I could only cling to God, my Creator and hold on tight. People told me they were praying for me and that was appreciated. Others sent cards that expressed their support.

I believe every person who is given a diagnosis of cancer thinks about the possibility of death, or the process of dying. Doctors try to answer the question, but the fact is, they really don't know. There are too many variables.

As patients we wonder if death is imminent and how we might experience it. Will it come quickly or drag out as we continue various treatments?

(Hospice is a wonderful service whose benefits come into play if it is expected that we will die within six months. The organization offers a variety of help to not only the patient, but the family as well.)

Is there another life somewhere that God created? Is that Heaven? Another Garden of Eden? Another planet? I believe Jesus was the Son of God who died for the sins of mankind. I believe the Holy Spirit exists to comfort and guide me. God's grace is available to anyone who asks the Lord to come into their life. Life eternal is the gift.

I now understand more about the Bible and am impressed with the history, and prophesies that came true centuries later.

If people don't believe in God as the Creator of life, then how do they view death? Will they know they died? Will their bodies turn to dust or ashes with no further knowledge or understanding—just--no more me? Are they here and then not here?

Paul writes in II Corinthians (Chapter 4:16-18)

"So, we're not giving up. How could we! Even though on the outside it often looks like things are falling apart on us, on the inside, where God is making new life, not a day goes by without his unfolding grace. These hard times are small potatoes compared to the coming good times, the lavish celebration prepared for us. There's far more here than meets the eye. The things we see now are here today, gone tomorrow. But the things we can't see now will last forever."

<u>The Message</u> (MSG) Copyright ©, 2002 by <u>Eugene H. Peterson</u>

I wonder about my family and how they would manage without me. I feel sad thinking about them. How long will it take for them to grieve and ultimately reach acceptance? What will they have learned from my time on earth?

When each of my boys was born, I had complete understanding and belief that God created this child. Humans would not have the knowledge or capability of producing such an intricate, miraculous being. Consider the brain and all the systems working in the body of a human. How awesome. Who on earth can adequately explain our universe and the rotation of the planets, realizing that there is much beyond our universe?

Cancer forces a person to define life--how it comes about and what to do with it. I never saw the cancer and barely felt the pea-sized tumor that contained the cancerous cells. I could have stopped the pills and IV's at any time, but I held a firm commitment to complete what had begun

I believe once a person comes to terms with death, they can face life one day at a time with much greater appreciation and determination.

When I began chemotherapy I asked the doctor to give me the lowest dose possible because my body doesn't tolerate strong substances. He said "not." We begin with the strongest dose and see what happens. What happened was that my white cells dictated a need to reduce the amount of drugs by 50%. That's what I told him!

I thought that as chemo went on, it would be easier. Not true. With each dose my body rebelled more. Weakness, concentration, blurry vision, difficulty with word retrieval and fatigue, took over. It seemed to me that I was looking through fog.

At the end of May I wanted to return to my work as an elementary school counselor at least for a week. I wanted to meet with the fifth graders to prepare them for the transition to middle school. I worked in two different buildings with a total of six classes of fifth grade students.

I will always remember when half-way through my presentation in one classroom a boy got out of his seat and was walking across the back of the room. When I inquired what he was doing (in my teacher voice) his response was that I looked so tired he was getting a chair for me.

Wow!   What an unexpected gift that I will always treasure.

July

It has been four months since I began chemotherapy. I am more than halfway through and feel relief and a sense of satisfaction. However, depression once again rises within me.

Now I fear that treatment for this cancer may never end or a new cancer might be discovered and start me on another course of chemotherapy.

July (IS IT CANCER?)

A cough, a sneeze. Is it normal?
  Or, is it a side-effect of chemotherapy?
  Or, is it CANCER?

A headache, different from others.
Is it sinus congestion or is it a side-effect   of
chemotherapy?
Or, is it CANCER?

A skin mole not of importance before the diagnosis of cancer, now it looks suspicious; yet, too petty to mention.

Still a worry. Is it CANCER?

Will I think this way the rest of my life?
Or, after chemotherapy ends, will I relax?

The unanswered question still remains--
did I have CANCER? Or do I have CANCER?

Note:

My internist managed my chemotherapy since it wasn't available anywhere in my small town, other than the hospital. I was able to drive myself to his office and back home and felt satisfied that I was receiving good care. One week he was going to be out of town and made arrangements for me to be infused at the hospital.

What happened was totally insane, considering that I had driven myself to the hospital. I had to put on a gown, get in bed and have an identification bracelet placed on my wrist. Someone went through my medical history with me. The nurse had trouble finding a vein – my left arm was used exclusively for blood work and chemotherapy because of the lymph nodes removed from under my armpit.

Hospital charges were ridiculous. The next time I saw my internist I gave him a list of complaints. Within several months he had hired someone to administer chemo drugs right there in his office.

I shared with him "Is it Cancer?"

His response was admirable. He simply said, "Show me the mole."

This was the second poem I had shared with him. He asked if I had more and if so he would like to see them. I proudly took to him the rest of what I had written.

Several days later he asked me to come in at the end of the day. We sat together and he told me the parts that were especially meaningful to him.

He was surprised at all the side-effects from chemotherapy I listed, saying that I had never shared those with him and some of them he had never heard from other patients. He told me I needed to publish what I had written and illustrated.

Then, he said something I have thought of often. "Now I must put my mantle back on in order to be your doctor." I understood. He had seen the inside and emotional parts of me that he couldn't treat so in order to remain objective he had to come back to his role as internist.

August (CHEMOTHERAPY MISERIES)

Chemo affected my TASTE, a metallic taste like aluminum foil. I did best when avoiding salt and spices. Watermelon was my favorite food.

Loud SOUND sent shivers up my back; especially loading and unloading the dishwasher, breaking ice cubes out of trays, even stirring sugar in iced tea.

TOUCH felt numb.

VISION was a major problem. It was like looking out through inner fog. Lights at night were florescent. Reading was a chore demanding great energy and concentration.

My SPEECH was slurred as I searched for words and struggled to organize my thoughts.

The MUSCLES at the surgery site tightened and cramped.

Chemotherapy caused me to go into menopause. My BODY TEMPERATURE jumped from shivering cold to volcanic style hot, off and on throughout the day and night.

And then the TIREDNESS – I couldn't lie down hard enough.

August   (THE SIXTH MONTH)

Yesterday I thought I was dying--
--dying of brain cancer
--as I awaited the results of a CT scan
--because of headaches that for two months now
come and go.

I know someone who just died of brain cancer.

Awaiting a diagnosis can seem an eternity.
Do I plan for next week, next month?
Is the future cancelled--or at least postponed?

Do I fear death, or do I fear losing life or the
quality of life to which I am accustomed?

Today (on a Sunday) my doctor called.
CT scan normal--cause of headaches unknown.

Headaches now seem unimportant. Cancer cells
are not the cause. Will this fear of cancer
continue forever, a curse I relentlessly bear?

Mid-August (THE SIXTH MONTH)

The end is in sight
Five months behind me, one ahead
Yet each time I say 'the end,' I fear.

I fear the possibility
--the possibility of cancer cells that I never knew were there,
--multiplying in my body unaffected by drugs, and, the possibility of a need for more chemotherapy.

I fear death by cancer--the possibility, a possibility I didn't accept earlier.

How can I feel excited or relieved about a last round when there are no guarantees that this will always be the last round?

September

The end of chemo did not return me to the person I was before the diagnosis of breast cancer. My hair was returning, but my energy was still a major problem. I had time to sit with a body that couldn't keep going and a mind that wouldn't stop going and a need for a sense of control.

Years ago my mother had given me a stitchery project that was waiting for needle and yarn. I began working on it and because the holes were large I could manage to get the needle through the holes. This I could control.

The picture was of penguins walking through a rainbow, black and white, becoming color, changing.

I too am changing.
I can never be the same.

Many years have passed since my diagnosis of breast cancer. The right side of my chest is an ever present reminder as I look at the scar.

Spiritual roots gave me something to hold on to when I struggled with control issues. Over and over I would submit to God, then back away and try to do things my way.

Had I focused my attention on Psalm 23, a psalm of David, it may have helped me get out of the control and depression issues. It would have benefitted me had I read this every day. I quote from the Contemporary English Version of the Bible. Used with permission of American Bible Society, Copyright © 1995

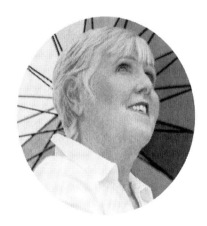

Psalm 23   THE GOOD SHEPHERD

"You, Lord, are my shepherd.
I will never be in need.
You let me rest in fields of green grass.

"You lead me to streams of peaceful water,
And you refresh my life.

"You are true to your name,
And you lead me
Along the right paths.
I may walk through valleys
As dark as death,
But I won't be afraid.

"You are with me,
And your shepherd's rod
makes me feel safe.

"You treat me to a feast,
While my enemies watch.
You honor me as your guest,

"And you fill my cup
Until it overflows.

"Your kindness and love
Will always be with me
Each day of my life,
And I will live forever
In your house, Lord"

POSTSCRIPT

We all know there is a chance of recurrence of cancer in the same area or another part of our body. Both Jack and Linda have lived with that truth.

In either case, we approach this new diagnosis with many of the same emotions. As far as treatment options we might find something new and a more accurate approach that can target the cancer.

Once again, knowledge and early diagnosis offer the patient the best chance of surviving and learning to live with cancer.

Alternative treatments have not been discussed in this book, but are widely available and should be researched.

Author's Website:

www.margaretbarnhart.com

email address: margeb730@cox.net

Personal Encounters with Cancer, 2016
      and

Journey Unknown, 2ⁿᵈ Edition, focusing
 on the emotional aspects of cancer,
mastectomy and chemotherapy, 2012

AVAILABLE FROM:

- ❖ My website above
- ❖ Amazon Print on Demand
- ❖ Amazon Kindle (there is an app for
   people without a Kindle Tablet)
- ❖ All bookstores

JOURNEY UNKNOWN TRIBUTES

Regarding *Journey Unknown, 2nd Edition, Focusing on the Emotional Aspects of Cancer, Mastectomy and Chemotherapy*

Nelda writes,

"In April, 2016, Encanterra Writing Club in Santay Valley, AZ, was very fortunate to discover Margaret. We wanted to find an author who would share his/her writing with us. She was a perfect fit and when the Book Club and Bible Study groups heard she was coming, they wanted to be included.

"The audience had different interests, but she kept all engrossed. She read portions of Journey Unknown—which are so well written they inspire, inform and give hope."

Bobbi writes regarding *Journey Unknown*,

"I loved Margaret's book. My only regret is that my sister died of breast cancer before having a chance to read it. I am giving it to her daughter."

Made in the USA
San Bernardino, CA
27 July 2016